Foam Roller
Techniques

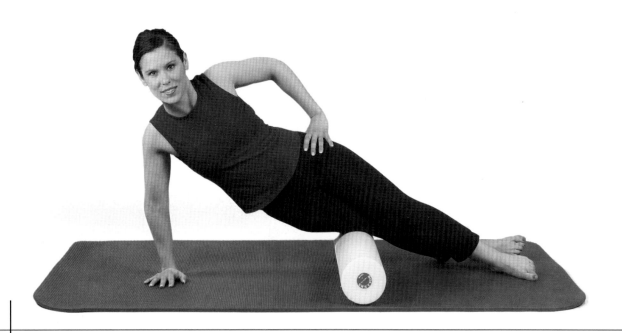

for massage, stretches and improved flexibility

Michael Fredericson, MD
Terri Lyn S. Yamamoto, PhD
Mark Fadil, CMT

Foam Roller Techniques

Contents

To order additional copies of Foam Roller Techniques contact OPTP (800) 367-7393 or www.optp.com.

First Edition. Printed in Minneapolis, MN
ISBN: 978-0-9764757-3-6

Introduction

To understand the benefits of using the foam roller for self-massage one can look to the benefits of massage in general. Self-massage using the foam roller is most comparable to deep tissue massage, myofascial release, and myofascial trigger point therapy. Regular treatments can increase flexibility, decrease muscle tension and pain, improve performance, and help prevent injury.

Massage is very effective at treating myofascial trigger points. These are taut bands, or knots, in muscle tissue that refer pain to other areas. For example, a trigger point in the gluteal muscle (at the outside of the hip) may refer pain down into the shin. In addition to pain, trigger points will also limit range-of-motion, inhibit muscle strength, and cause early muscle fatigue. You can treat a trigger point by applying pressure directly to the taut band of muscle that causes the referred pain. As you hold on the spot you should notice the referred pain start to go away. Consistent treatments can completely eliminate the painful trigger point and help restore normal muscle function.

Massage is also effective at mobilizing soft tissue such as muscles, neural tissue, fascia, and tendons. It's similar to stretching, but because you're applying pressure to an isolated area, you're able to focus the mobilization on a specific spot. This is useful for treating knots or bands of tight muscle, breaking adhesions within and between muscles and fascia, and accessing areas that are difficult to treat with conventional stretches. The end result is increased flexibility and more normal movement patterns.

Regular massage can also help detect when muscles are starting to tighten. When your muscles are loose, massage should be relatively pain free. As adhesions develop, and your muscles tighten, the tissue becomes more sensitive and massage becomes more painful. If you're using massage on a regular basis, you can catch changes early based on how you feel during treatments. You may notice that an area starts to get painful during massage before you notice much tightness or pain during your activities. This indicates that you need to focus more attention on the tight area until it becomes less painful. This approach will help prevent small problems from turning into something more serious.

How to Use the Foam Roller

To maximize the effectiveness of the foam roller we recommend making it a part of your daily stretching routine. You should use the roller before and after activity, and always roll before you stretch. This will help to warm up cold muscles and prepare them for deeper and more aggressive stretching. It also enforces normal movement patterns after the tissue has been mobilized.

Make sure you only roll on soft tissue and do not roll over joints, ligaments, or bony protrusions. Start by placing your body on the roller and slowly roll up and down the muscle indicated. If you find a knot or tight band, hold that spot and try to feel the tissue release and soften underneath the pressure. As you hold, take deep breaths and try to keep your body as relaxed as possible. If the area does not release after one minute continue rolling other areas and try again later.

Self-massage using the foam roller can be painful. This is an indication that the area is tight and needs attention. If an area's too painful to roll, place your body on the roller for 10 - 15 seconds before moving on to a new spot. As the tissue starts to loosen up you should be able to roll with less pain. In the following exercises we have indicated ways to minimize and maximize the amount of pressure you can apply when rolling. Start by using less pressure and gradually increase as your muscles begin to loosen.

Certain areas are more likely to become bruised or sore with aggressive treatment. (We will point out these areas throughout the book.) If you do become bruised or sore from using the roller you have gone too deep or too long. Do not roll again until the bruises have cleared, and begin again with less pressure. Remember, it's always better to be cautious than to go too deep and risk tissue damage.

We have tried to limit each area of the body to one or two pages. Several variations of each exercise are shown followed by two or three stretches. Start by doing the easiest version of the exercise and progress as you become comfortable. For the most effective stretch, slowly position yourself and gradually increase the tension until you begin to feel a "good" uncomfortable stretch. Hold the position until you feel the tissue begin to release. (This may take 20 - 60 seconds.) Never stretch to the point of pain or irritation and don't hold your stretch for more than 60 seconds. After you feel the tissue give, release the stretch and repeat with a further limitation. Do not exceed four repetitions.

We hope you find all the exercises and stretches to be effective and easy-to-follow. Happy rolling!

Upper Neck

suboccipital, neck extensors

Small Ball Massage

● Tools Needed: Small Ball, 36" x 4" Foam Roller, Stability Ball

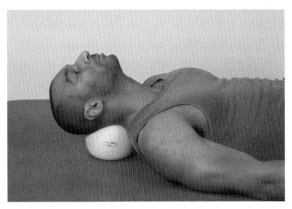

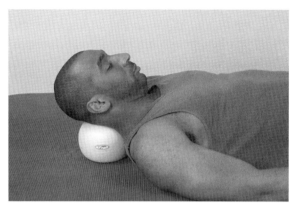

Gently lie on your back and place a massage ball between the base of your skull and top of your neck. Allow your entire neck region, and body, to relax.

Slowly nod your head forward and back allowing the upper neck muscles to further relax and settle into the ball. Use different sized balls to vary the focus and intensity of the massage.

Foam Roller Variation

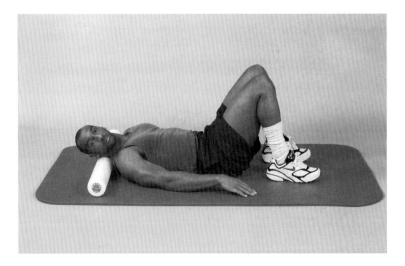

The foam roller can be used as an alternative to the massage described above if you do not have access to massage balls.

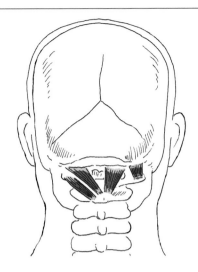

Begin by sitting on a stability ball, or in a chair. Keeping your spine upright and shoulders down, place your hand behind your head and tilt your chin forward until a stretch is felt throughout the back of your neck.

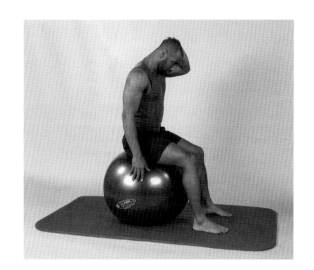

Stretches

Stand or sit upright. Keeping your spine straight and still, press your head forward jutting your chin out as far as possible.

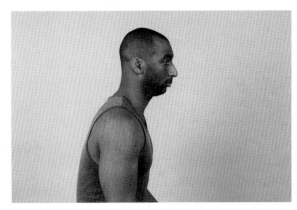

Slowly reverse the movement pulling your head back as far as possible. Your head should stay level throughout the movement. You should feel a stretch at the base of your neck.

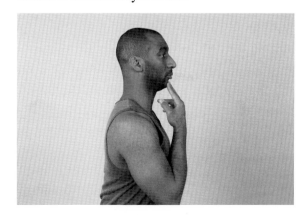

2

Lower Neck

levator scapulae, upper trapezius, scalenes, sternocleidomastoid

Small Ball Massage

Tools Needed: Small Ball

Gently lie on your back and place a massage ball at the side and slightly to the back of your neck. Relax and let your head and neck settle. Slightly tuck your chin in toward your chest to lengthen your neck, and continue to settle into the ball. Repeat on the other side.

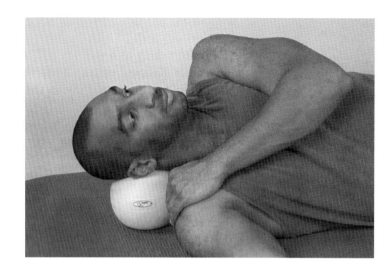

Variations

Vary the massage described above by changing the rotation of your head to target different areas of your neck. Address any areas of tightness.

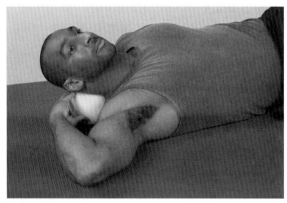

To intensify the massage, lift your hips off the floor to distribute more pressure to the region being massaged. Repeat on the other side.

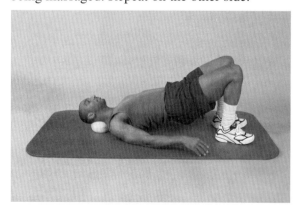

Exercises

levator scapulae, upper trapezius, scalenes, sternocleidomastoid

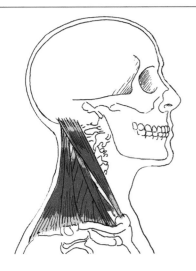

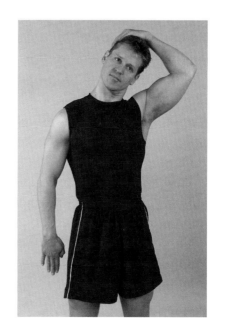

The focus of this stretch is on the upper trapezius. Looking straight ahead, lower your left ear toward your left shoulder while keeping your right shoulder depressed and your right arm reaching down. Use your left hand to assist in lowering your head for a deeper stretch along the side of your neck. Repeat on the other side.

Note: All of these stretches can be performed while sitting. This allows you to hook your arm under the side of a chair to help anchor the shoulder.

Stretches

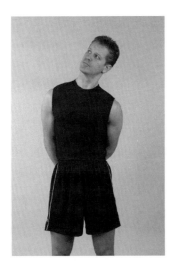

The focus of this stretch is on the scalenes. Tilt your head sideways toward your left shoulder. With your left hand, clasp your right wrist and gently pull your right arm down toward your body's midline. While maintaining this stretch, rotate your head slightly up toward the ceiling. A stretch should be felt along the front, right side of the neck. Repeat on the opposite side.

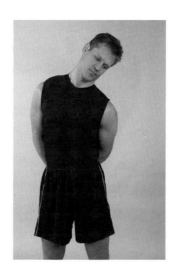

The focus of this stretch is on the levator scapulae. Tilt your head sideways toward your left shoulder. With your left hand, clasp your right wrist and gently pull your right arm down toward your body's midline. While maintaining this stretch, rotate your head slightly down toward the ground. A stretch should be felt from the back, base of your skull down to the back of your right shoulder. Repeat on the opposite side.

4

Posterior and Lateral Shoulder

serratus anterior, posterior capsule, lateral/rear deltoids

Foam Roller Stretch

● Tools Needed: 36"x 6" Foam Roller

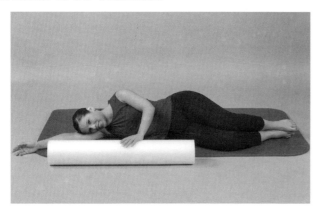

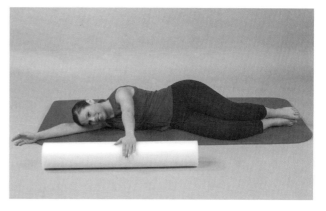

Start side-lying as depicted in the photos. Extend your right arm and place the palm of your left hand on the roller. Keeping your hips stacked and torso still, push the roller out and back extending and retracting through the shoulder and shoulder blades.

As your shoulder muscles relax, increase the range-of-motion for a greater stretch. Repeat on the opposite side.

Variation

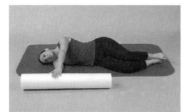

1.

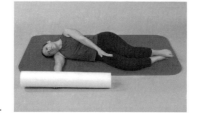

2.

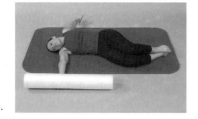

3.

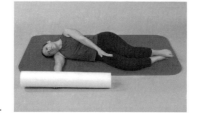

4.

Start side-lying with the foam roller placed in front of you and parallel to your body. Keeping your hips stacked and lower torso still, reach your left arm out over the foam roller. Keeping the extension in your left arm, slowly circle your arm over, back, and around while attempting to brush your finger tips along the floor as you circle. You'll feel a stretch through the entire shoulder region. Repeat on the opposite side.

Exercises

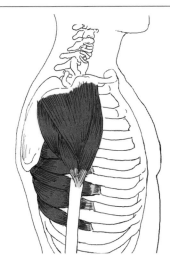

The focus of this stretch is on the lateral deltoid. Stand upright with your shoulders pressed down. Keeping your right arm straight, fold it across your chest with your palms facing in. Avoid rotating your shoulders or trunk. With your left arm press lightly on the fore-arm or upper arm (not the elbow) until a stretch is felt at the back of the shoulder. To focus on the rear deltoid, lift your right arm toward your chin. Repeat on the other side.

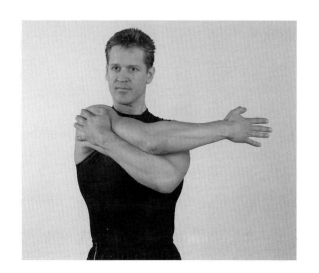

Stretches

This stretch is for the posterior shoulder capsule. Start lying on your right side and extend your right arm in front of your torso bending the elbow 90 degrees. Keeping your shoulder and upper arm on the ground, press your right arm down with your left hand until a stretch is felt at the back of the shoulder.

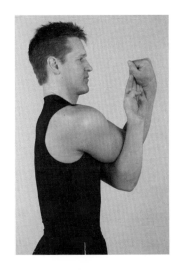

This stretch is for your right side. In a standing position cross your right elbow over your left arm. Clasp your hands and slowly raise both arms while maintaining a neutral head position, and without letting your shoulders rise. You'll feel a stretch in the right rear shoulder region. Repeat on the opposite side.

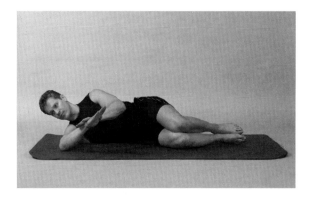

Lateral Chest

latissimus dorsi, teres major

Foam Roller Massage

● Tools Needed: 36" x 6" Foam Roller

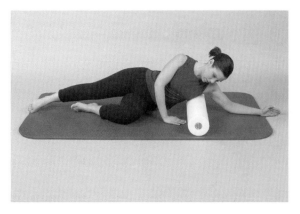

Start lying on your left side with the foam roller below your armpit and positioned perpendicular to your body. Lean back slightly and extend your left arm out with your palm facing forward.

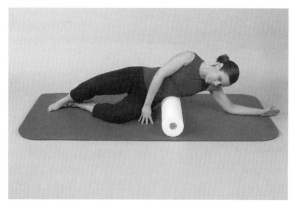

Using your right arm for leverage, roll the lateral upper torso along the foam roller. Repeat on the opposite side.

Foam Roller Stretches

Outstretch your arms placing your palms on the foam roller. Sit back on your heels with toes folded under. Focus on stretching forward rather than down. A stretch should be felt along the side of your upper back.

To intensify the stretch, bend your arms and place your elbows on the foam roller.

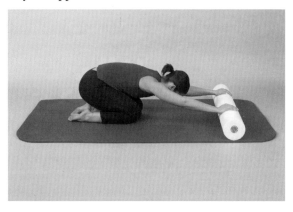

● **Note:** Be careful not to hyperextend your shoulders by letting them drop down toward the floor.

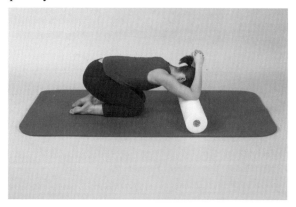

Exercises

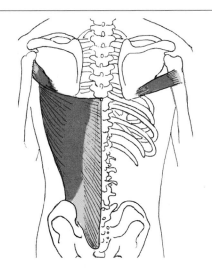

Begin by kneeling. Outstretch your arms and place them onto a stability ball or chair. Slowly lower down onto your heels. Widen your back by drawing your shoulder blades apart and turning your thumbs up. Focus on reaching forward rather than sinking down.

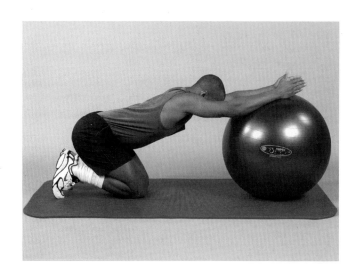

Stretches

Begin by kneeling. Lower down onto your heels and extend your right arm overhead and slightly to the left. Shift your hips to the right to intensify the stretch through the right side of your upper back. Repeat on the left side.

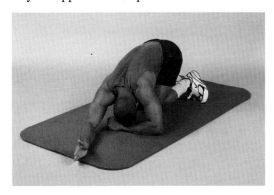

Start on your hands and knees with your left arm outstretched in front of you. Weave your right arm under your left armpit and reach out as far as possible keeping your palm facing up. Bend your left arm and allow your upper trunk to rotate until you feel a stretch through the back of your right shoulder. Repeat on the left side.

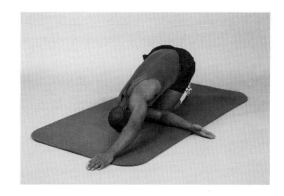

8

Upper Back

rhomboids, middle trapezius, thoracic spine

Foam Roller Massage

⬤ Tools Needed: 36" x 6" Foam Roller

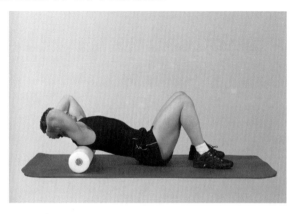

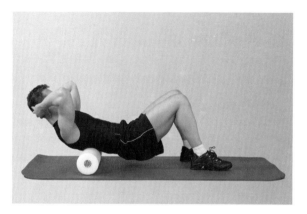

Lie with the foam roller under your upper back. Place your hands behind your head with your elbows drawn in slightly toward midline– this allows your shoulder blades to separate.

Draw your belly button in and lift your hips up off the floor using your legs for leverage. Roll up and down on the roller from your shoulders down to the bottom of your rib cage.

Foam Roller Stretch

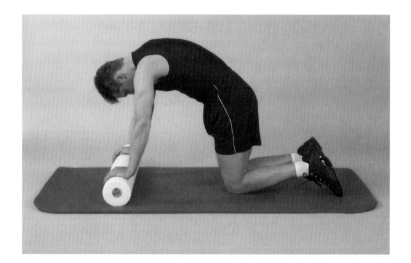

Start in quadruped position with your hands placed on the foam roller. Round your back tucking your chin into your chest and tailbone under. Raise your upper back until a stretch is felt in that region.

Exercises

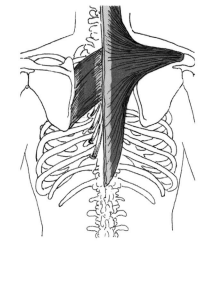

Start kneeling and place your hands under your lower legs. Drop your head and slowly start to round your back allowing your arms to straighten. You should feel a stretch through your upper back.

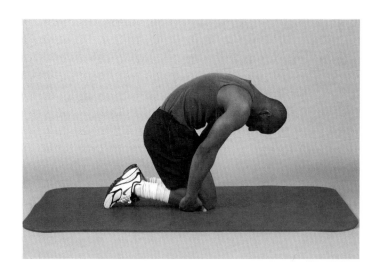

Start on all fours in a quadruped position. Place one hand on the back of your head. Keeping your spine straight, and hips level, slowly rotate your upper torso toward the ceiling and then back down toward the floor.

Continue with this movement and gradually increase your range-of-motion for added stretch. Repeat on the other side.

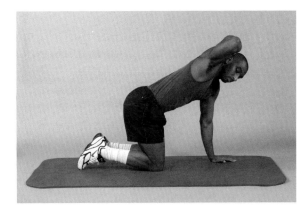

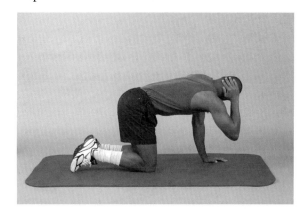

Stretches

10

Anterior Chest

pectorals, subscapularis, anterior deltoid

Foam Roller Stretch

● Tools Needed: 36" x 6" Foam Roller

Lie with your spine inline with the foam roller. Be sure to keep your head and hips supported on the roller. Keeping your shoulders pressed toward your feet, stretch your arms out to the side with your palms facing up. Relax into the foam roller allowing the front of your chest to stretch.

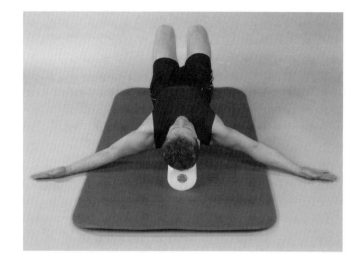

● **Note:** Be careful not to arch your back.

Variation

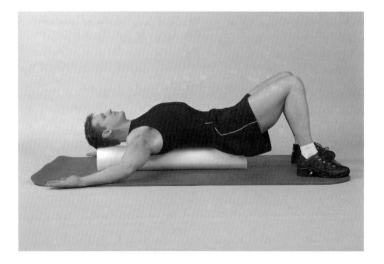

Lie with your spine inline with the foam roller. Be sure to keep your head and hips supported on the roller. Keeping your shoulders pressed toward your feet, stretch your arms out to the side with your palms facing up. Bend your elbows about 90 degrees and try to touch the floor with the backs of your hands. Relax into the foam roller allowing the front of your chest to stretch. Be careful not to arch your back.

Exercises

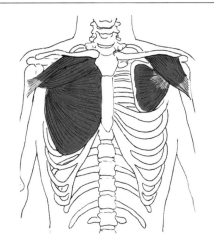

The focus of this stretch is on the chest. Reach your arms out to the side forming a 90 degree bend at the elbows. Without arching your back, and without letting your head extend forward, bring your arms back until a stretch is felt through the front of your chest. For an increased stretch, place your forearms on the back edge of a doorframe and press your chest forward.

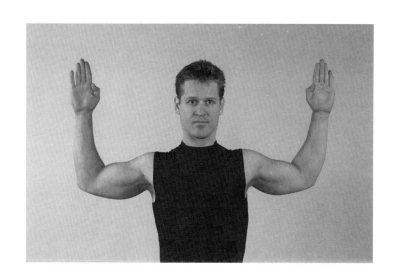

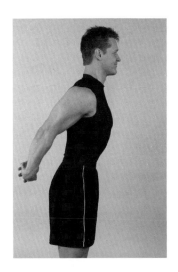

Clasp your hands together behind your back and depress your shoulders. Extend your arms back and gradually draw them upward until you feel a stretch through the front of your chest, or until you reach your end range-of-motion. Be sure to maintain an upright position with your head in a neutral position.

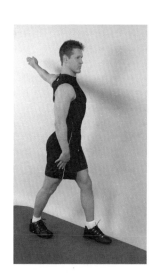

Stand sideways with your left side facing a wall. Extend your left arm behind and place your palm against the wall while keeping your shoulders down and back. Slowly turn your body away from the wall keeping your extended arm in contact with the wall. Repeat on the opposite side.

Stretches

Foam Roller Stretch

⬤ Tools Needed: 36" x 6" Foam Roller

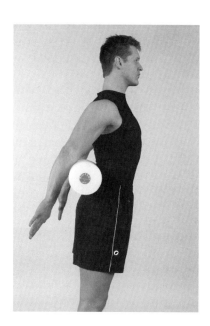

While standing, place the foam roller behind your lower back and secure it by extending your arms over it. Stand in an upright position and push the foam roll into your lower back. Repeat the stretch focusing on different areas of your lower back. Be careful not to over stretch.

Variation

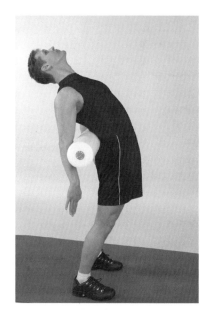

To intensify the stretch, gently arch backwards over the foam roller while drawing your arms forward for leverage.

Exercises

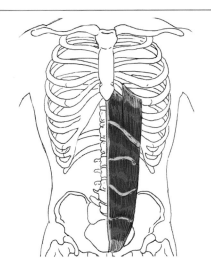

Start by lying face down on the floor. Keeping your gluteals relaxed and hips pressed to the floor, place your hands below your shoulders and draw your chest forward and up while keeping your shoulders away from your ears. Slowly extend upward until you feel a stretch in the front of your mid-section.

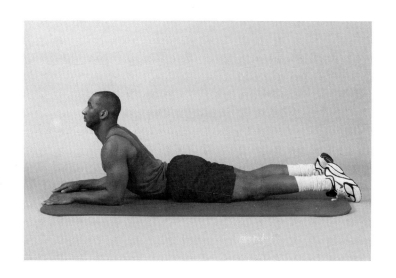

Stretches

Start upright in a kneeling position. Place your hands on your lower back and press your shoulders down. Draw your elbows and shoulder blades together. Lift your chest up and slowly arch your back beginning at the upper chest. Press your hips forward.

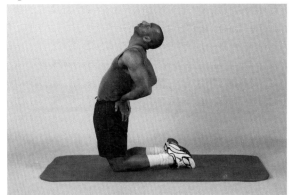

To intensify the stretch, reach back and place your hands on your heels. Start with your toes curled under and progress to performing the stretch with the tops of your feet against the floor.

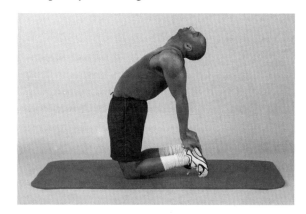

14

Lower Back

lumbar extensor muscles

Foam Roller Massage

● Tools Needed: 36" x 6" Foam Roller

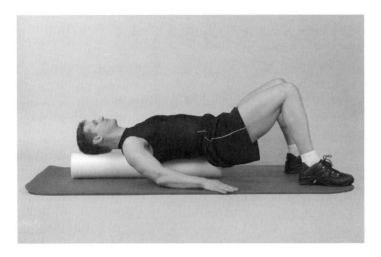

Position the roller so that it's inline with your spine. To focus on your right side, roll your body to the left, keeping your spine parallel to the roller, and stop on the muscles that run along the length of your spine. Hold and allow to relax. Repeat on the left side.

Variation

Position the foam roller horizontally along your lower back. Gently roll back and forth, stopping in tight areas to allow your spine to relax.

● Caution, avoid this variation if you have lower back issues.

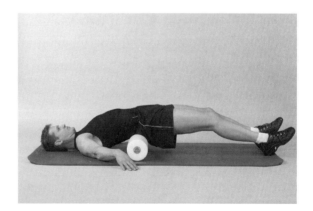

Exercises

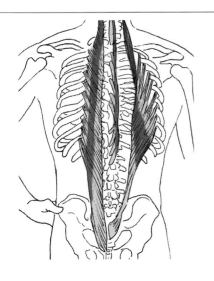

Bend your right leg and cross it over your left thigh. Place your left arm across your right thigh. Roll your hips forward to keep your spine upright and rotate your spine gradually to the right using your back muscles and left arm for leverage. Turn your head to the right as you rotate. Repeat on the other side.

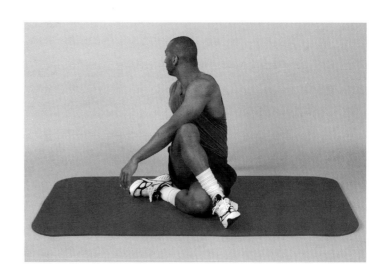

Stretches

Start in a quadruped position with your hands placed directly under your shoulders. Drop your head, tuck your chin to your chest, and shift your tailbone under while rounding your back.

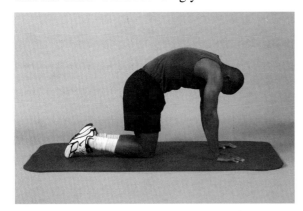

Next, roll your hips forward, arch your back, draw your shoulder blades together, and look up. Repeat several times to mobilize your lower back from flexion to extension of the spine.

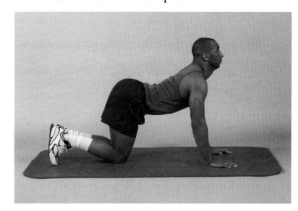

16

obliques, quadratus lumborum muscle

Foam Roller Massage

● Tools Needed: 36" x 6" Foam Roller

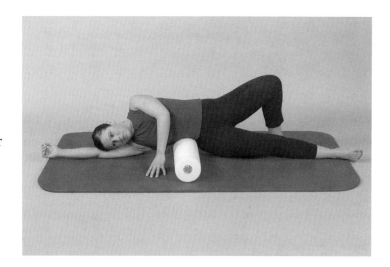

Position yourself as shown placing the foam roller between your ribs and hip. Slowly roll backwards until you feel a stretch and pressure in your lower back region. Hold on tight spots until you feel the tissue soften. Do not hold on any one spot for longer than a minute. Be careful not to over-treat. Repeat on the opposite side.

● **Note:** If pain is felt radiating down your leg stop exercise *immediately.*

Variation

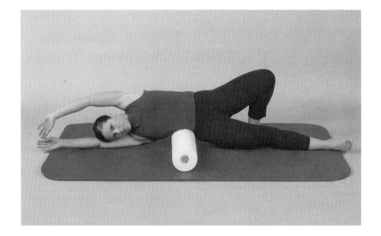

To increase the intensity of the massage raise your left arm overhead. Carefully ease into the massage to protect your low back. Repeat on the opposite side.

Exercises

obliques, quadratus lumborum muscle

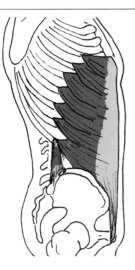

Start by standing or kneeling in an upright position. Extend your right arm up overhead as your left arm reaches down toward the floor. Holding the extension, lower your right arm over to the left and slightly forward until a stretch is felt through your right side and back. Repeat the stretch on the left side.

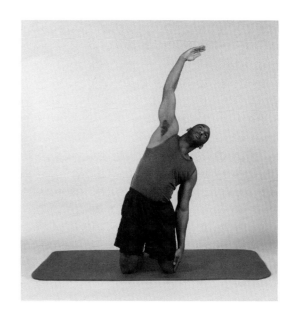

Stretches

Lie on your back with your left leg extended. Bring your right knee to your chest and extend your right arm to the side at shoulder level. Slowly lower your right leg across your torso keeping both shoulders on the floor. Repeat on the other side.

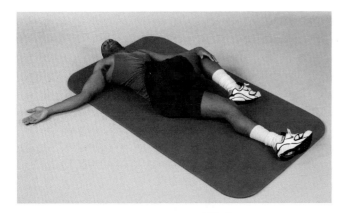

Sit in a half-straddle position with your right leg bent and the left straight. Grasp your left leg and extend the right arm overhead while bending to the left. Keep your shoulders relaxed and turn your head up toward your overhead arm. Avoid spinal rotation and keep both hips anchored to the floor. Repeat on the opposite side.

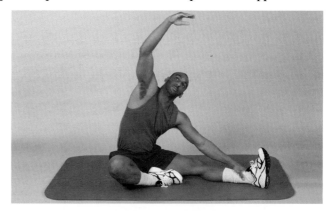

triceps, biceps

Foam Roller Massage

⬤ Tools Needed: 36" x 6" Foam Roller, Stretch Out® Strap

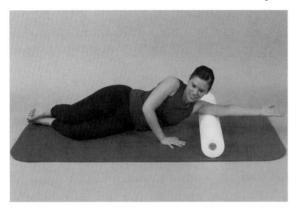

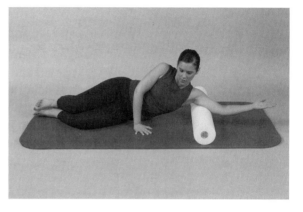

With the roller perpendicular to your body, extend your left arm and place the roller on the backside of your upper arm. For leverage, place your right arm out in front of your torso.

Roll your left arm along the roller to massage the backside (tricep) of that arm. To vary the massage, bend your left elbow and then proceed. Repeat on the opposite side.

Foam Roller Stretch

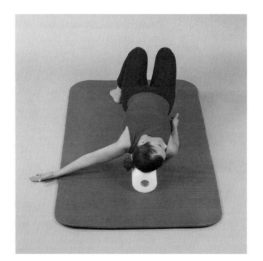

Lie on the roller so that it's inline with your spine. Be sure that your head is supported. Extend your left arm out perpendicular to your body with your palm facing up. Slowly rotate your head and torso to the right until a stretch is felt along the front of the left upper arm (bicep). Repeat on the right side.

Exercises

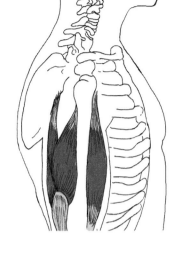

The focus of this stretch is on the triceps and front of the shoulder. Start in a standing position and grasp the Stretch Out® Strap with your right hand. With the strap in hand, bring your right arm up slightly behind your head. Draw your left shoulder forward and bring your left arm behind your back. Grasp the opposite end of the strap and inch your hands together while maintaining a neutral head position. Repeat on the opposite side.

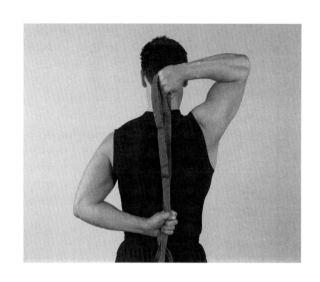

Stretches

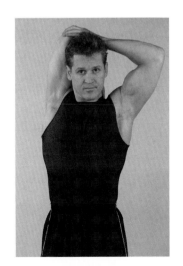

The focus of this stretch is on the triceps. Start standing and extend your right arm behind your head with elbow bent. Use your left hand to deepen the stretch by pulling your elbow further back. Repeat on the opposite side.

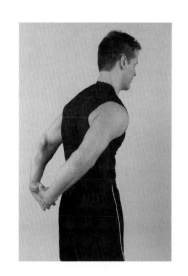

The focus of this stretch is on the biceps. Start standing and reach behind your back and interlace your fingers. Keeping your back straight and shoulders depressed, invert your hands so that your palms are facing down. Slowly lift your arms up.

20

Exercises

Half Foam Roller Stretches

Tools Needed: 12" x 3" Half Foam Roller

The focus of this stretch is on the wrist extensors. Start on your knees and place the tops of your hands onto a half foam roller with your arms straight and fingers facing toward you. Slowly lower back on your heels while keeping your hands on the foam roller. A stretch should be felt through the top of your lower arms and wrists.

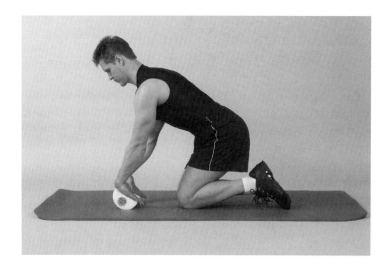

Variation

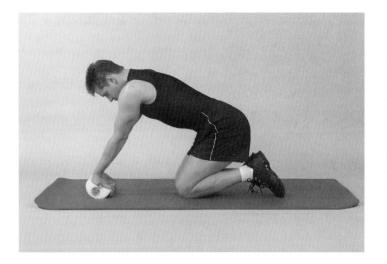

The focus of this stretch is on the wrist flexors and forearms. Start on your knees by placing your palms on a half foam roller. Keeping your arms straight, turn your palms under with your fingers facing toward you. Slowly lower back onto your heels while keeping your hands on the roller. A stretch should be felt through your wrists and forearms.

21

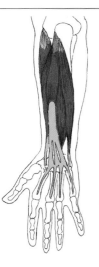

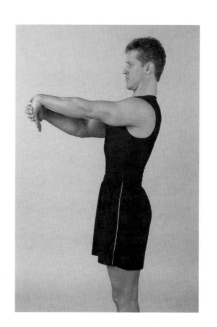

The focus of this stretch is on the wrist extensors. Keeping your left arm straight, and palm facing you, fold the palm of your left hand downward. Using your right hand, gently increase the bend in your wrist by pressing your hand toward your forearm. Repeat on the opposite side.

Note: Slightly rotating your wrist in either direction will intensify the stretch.

Stretches

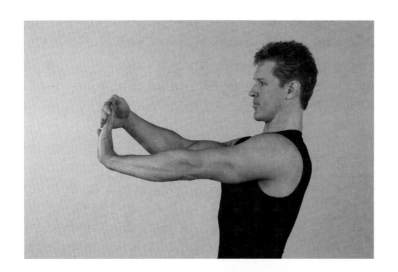

The focus of this stretch is on the wrist flexors and forearms. Extend your left arm (be sure to keep it straight) with palm facing out. Using your right hand, gently bend your wrist by pulling toward your body. Repeat on the opposite side.

Foam Roller Massage

⬤ Tools Needed: 36" x 6" Foam Roller

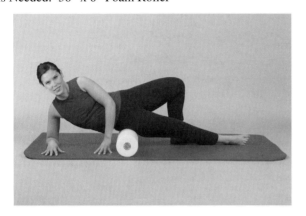

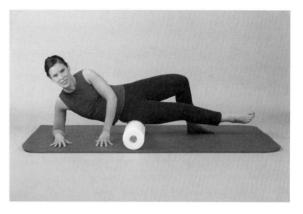

Start side-lying on the foam roller. Extend your right leg so that it's inline with your torso and rotate back to position your right gluteal on the roller. Bend and place your left leg behind your right, and place both hands on the floor for support.

Proceed to roll the right gluteal region along the roller. Repeat for your left side.

Variation

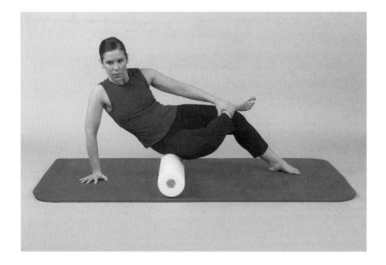

To intensify the stretch, bend and cross your right leg over your left thigh shifting your weight into the right gluteal region. Using your left leg for leverage, roll the right gluteal region along the foam roller. Adjust your rotation to find tight areas. For an added stretch, draw your left knee toward your right shoulder. Repeat for the left side.

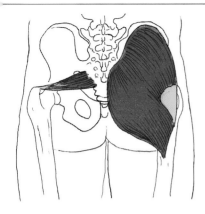

This stretch is for the right gluteal region. Bend your right knee and turn it out to about 2 O'Clock from center. (Be sure that your weight is evenly distributed between your hips.) Slowly fold your torso over your bent right knee. To vary the stretch, shift your upper body to each side or vary your knee angle up to 90 degrees. Repeat on the opposite side.

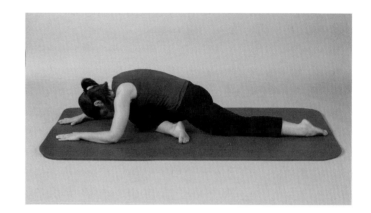

Stretches

For the right gluteal region, place your left leg on a chair or against a wall for support. Cross your lower right leg over your left thigh. Your right hand can be used to push your right knee further away from your torso to intensify the stretch.

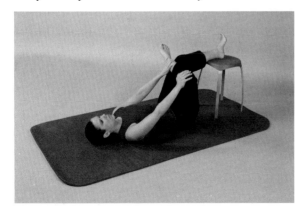

As you become more comfortable, try the stretch without support. For added intensity, pull your left thigh toward your left shoulder and lift your head off the floor. Use your right elbow to press your right knee away from your torso. Repeat for the opposite side.

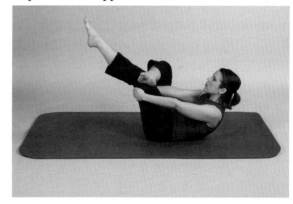

Foam Roller Massage

● Tools Needed: 36" x 6" Foam Roller

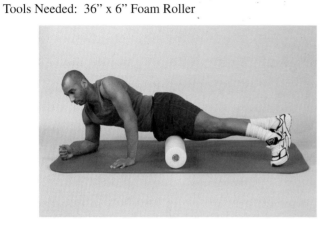

Lie down placing the front portion of your right hip (where the hip creases) on the roller. Extend your left leg and place your toes on the floor to help lift your left hip up off the roller.

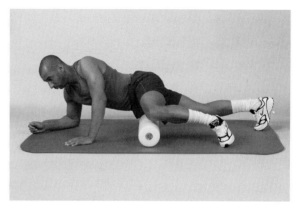

Keeping your left foot on the ground, slowly bend and straighten your left leg to roll your right hip along the roller. Repeat on the opposite side.

Variation

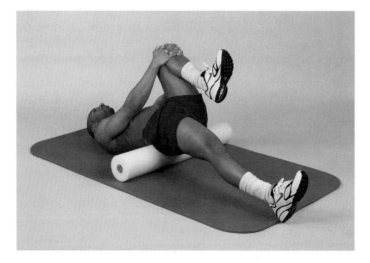

Place the foam roller under your hips. Be careful not to arch your lower back. Pull your left knee up to your chest and allow your right leg to relax and straighten. Push the bottom of your pelvis up toward the ceiling until a stretch is felt through the front of your right hip. Repeat on the opposite side.

Exercises

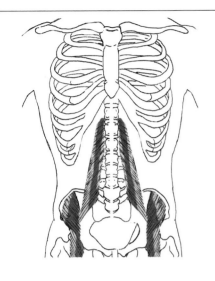

This stretch is shown for the right hip flexor. Start lying on you left side with both knees bent and your head resting on your left arm. With your right hand, clasp your right ankle or foot. Pinch your buttocks together and slowly tuck your tailbone under until a stretch is felt in the front of the right hip. Explore the stretch by varying the degree of pelvic tilt. Repeat on the opposite side.

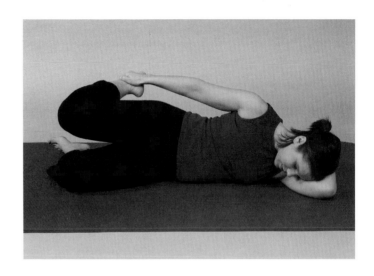

Stretches

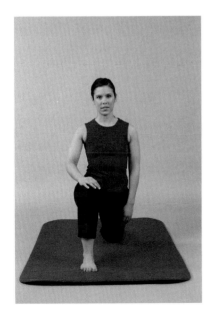

This stretch is for the left hip flexor. Start in a kneeling position with your right leg forward. Make sure your right knee doesn't extend past your ankle. Pinch your buttocks together and point your knees inward. Tuck your tailbone under until a stretch is felt at the top of your left thigh.

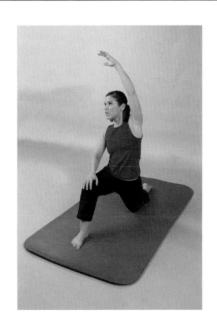

To enhance the stretch, reach your left arm up and bend your torso to the right. Be careful not to lean forward or backward. Repeat on the opposite side.

Upper Legs

tensor fascia latae, illotibial band

Foam Roller Massage

● Tools Needed: 36" x 6" Foam Roller, Stretch Out® Strap

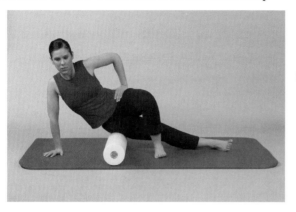

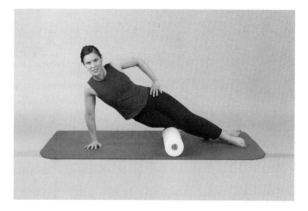

● **Note:**
This may be painful at first, so be sure to perform this massage in moderation.

Start side-lying on your right side with the roller just below your hip bone. Bend your left leg and place it in front of your right leg. With your right leg extended and inline with your torso, lift your right foot a few inches off the floor.

While maintaining a neutral head position, keeping your ear aligned with your shoulder, use your left leg for leverage and roll along your outer thigh from the bottom of your hip bone to just above your knee. (Do not roll over knee joint.) Repeat on the opposite side.

Variation

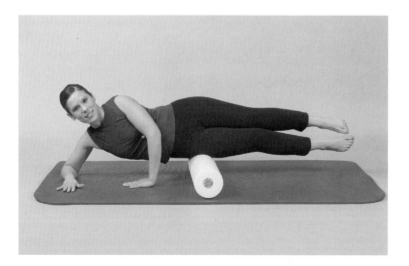

To intensify the massage, lift both legs off the floor and proceed to roll along the foam roller as described above. This is a very intense massage, be careful not to overdo it.

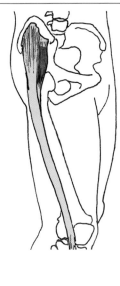

Place the Stretch Out® Strap around your right foot and secure the opposite end with your left hand. Extend your right arm out to the side for stability. Gently pull on the strap and allow your right leg to cross over to the left until a stretch is felt along the outer right thigh. Be sure to keep your right hip on the floor and do not hyper-extend your right knee. Repeat on the opposite side.

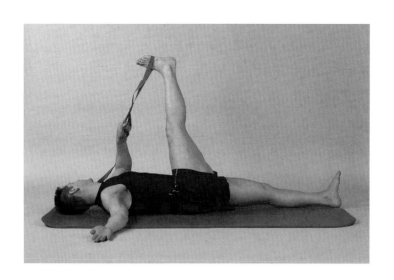

Stretches

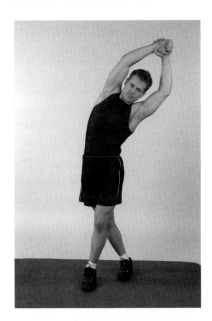

Begin standing and place your right leg behind your left bending your left knee slightly. Keeping your torso facing forward, clasp your right wrist with your left hand and draw your right arm up diagonally while pressing your right hip out. A stretch should be felt along the right outer thigh. Repeat on the opposite side.

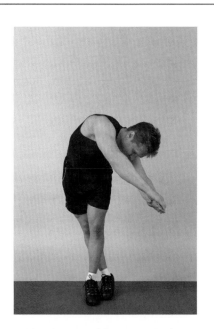

To vary the stretch, clasp and extend your arms. Bend down diagonally to your left and slightly bend your right knee. Repeat on the opposite side.

Note:
If you feel a stretch more in your hamstrings they're probably tight, take a moment to stretch them and then resume.

quadriceps

Foam Roller Massage

⬤ Tools Needed: 36" x 6" Foam Roller, Stretch Out® Strap

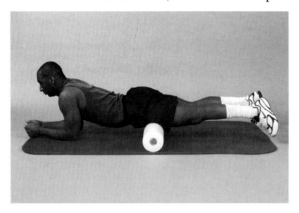

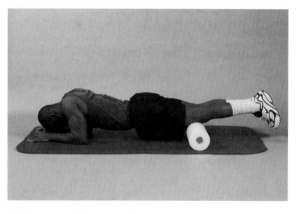

Position the foam roller under your quadriceps. Support your weight on your forearms and keep your belly button drawn in toward your spine to protect your lower back.

Using your forearms for leverage, roll from the bottom of your hip to the top of your knees. To intensify, lift a leg off the roller and do one at a time. Explore the stretch by rolling on both the inner and outer surfaces of your quadriceps.

Variation

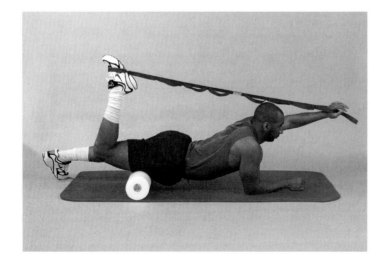

For a more focused massage, loop the Stretch Out® Strap around the foot of the leg to be massaged and roll along the quadricep. You can vary the intensity of the stretch by increasing or decreasing the tension on the strap. Repeat on the other side.

Exercises

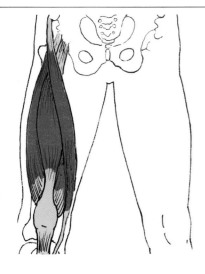

Start kneeling with your left leg in front. (Place padding under your back knee if desired.) Loop the Stretch Out® Strap around your right foot and slowly draw the strap forward using arm strength only. A stretch should be felt in your right quadricep. Be careful not to arch your lower back. Repeat on the opposite side.

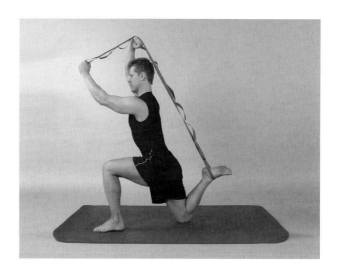

Clasp your right foot with one or two hands. (Use a wall or piece of furniture for support, if needed.) Keep your right thigh parallel to your left and push the bottom of your pelvis forward to intensify the stretch. To vary the stretch, pull your right foot across and away from your body. Repeat on the opposite side.

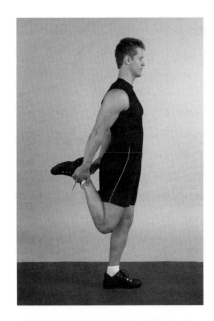

Begin by kneeling with your left leg in front. Grasp your right foot and pull it up toward your buttocks while pushing the bottom of your pelvis forward. To focus on the inner quadricep, pull your foot slightly out to the right side. Repeat on the opposite side.

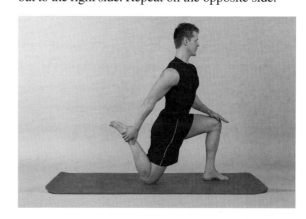

Stretches

30

Foam Roller Massage

⬤ Tools Needed: 36" x 6" Foam Roller, Stretch Out® Strap

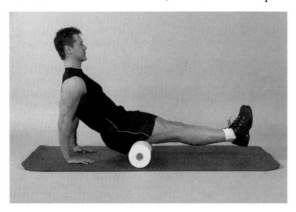

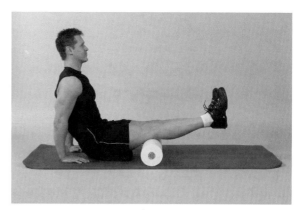

Position your hamstrings on the roller and lean back slightly using your arms to support your weight. With hips and heels off the floor, use your arms for leverage and roll along your hamstrings from the bottom of your hip bone to the top of your knees.

Do not roll over the back of your knees. Slightly rotate your legs to each side to massage the outer surfaces of your hamstrings. To intensify, bend forward at the hips (as shown).

Variation

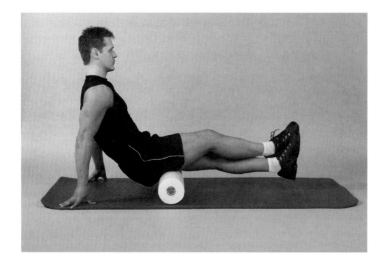

For a deeper massage, position yourself as described above, but this time with your right leg crossed over your left. Intensify the massage by pushing down with your top leg. Repeat on the opposite side.

Exercises

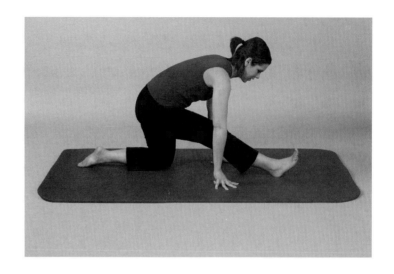

Start kneeling with your right leg extended forward (straight, but not locked) with your toes pulled back. Keeping your back straight, bend forward at the hip placing your arms to the sides for support. Rotate your torso to the left or right to emphasize the outer or inner hamstring, respectively. Point your toes forward and away from you to vary the location of the stretch along the hamstring. Repeat on the left side.

On your back, place the Stretch Out® Strap on the arch of your right foot. Extend your right leg up and left leg out. With toes flexed, hips anchored, and knees straight (not locked) draw your right leg toward your torso. A stretch should be felt along your right hamstring. Repeat on the opposite side.

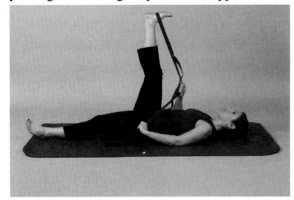

Start with your right thigh against your chest with right knee bent. Place the Stretch Out® Strap on the arch of your right foot and pull in toward your torso. Keep your right thigh against your chest and gradually straighten your leg until a stretch is felt along the upper hamstring.

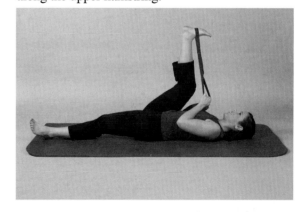

Stretches

inner thighs (adductors)

Foam Roller Massage

⬤ Tools Needed: 36" x 6" Foam Roller, Stretch Out® Strap

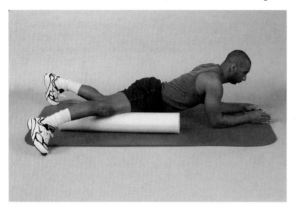

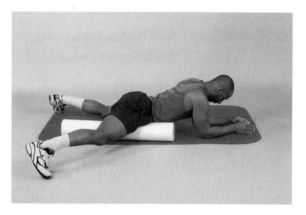

Place the foam roller on the inner thigh of your right leg keeping your hips open and right leg turned out slightly. Place your forearms on the floor for support and lift your hips off the floor.

Roll up and down in various planes using your arms and left leg for leverage. Be careful when rolling near the muscle origins at the hip creases, these areas may be sensitive. Repeat on the left side.

Modification

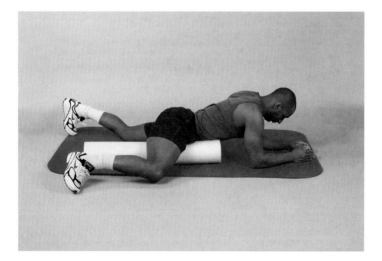

If flexibility is an issue, keep your right leg bent while performing the massage. Repeat on the other side.

Exercises

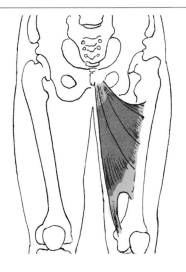

Begin by sitting against a wall and place the soles of your feet together. Bring your heels in toward your body and lightly press down on your knees with your hands. Keeping your back straight, gently open your knees toward the floor stretching the inner thigh (adductor) muscles. Place your elbows against your inner knees to increase the stretch. To vary this stretch, place your hands either on your ankles or lower legs. Avoid pulling up on your feet during the stretch.

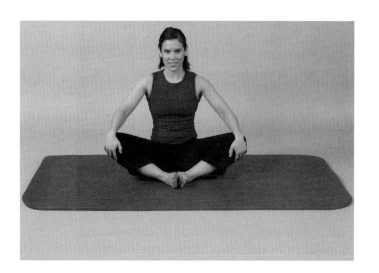

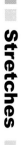

Start with your feet wide apart and lower down by bending your left leg. Keeping your back straight and hips level and square, ease down to stretch your right inner thigh. Repeat for the left side. (If stretch is too difficult, perform in a more upright position using a chair for support.)

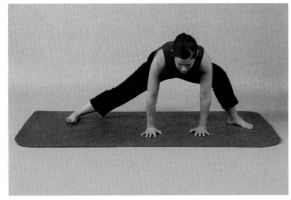

Wrap the Stretch Out® Strap around your right foot and lower your leg away from your body. Be sure to keep your left hip anchored to the floor. To intensify the stretch along the inside of your thigh, pull on the strap to lower your leg. Vary the stretch by pointing your toes in and out. Repeat on the opposite side.

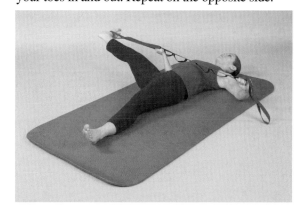

Lower Legs

calf (gastrocnemium & soleus)

Foam Roller Massage

⬤ Tools Needed: 36" x 6" Foam Roller, OPTP Slant™

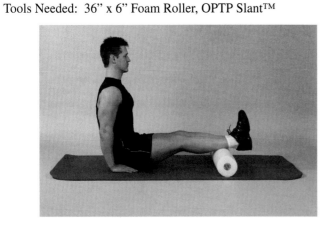

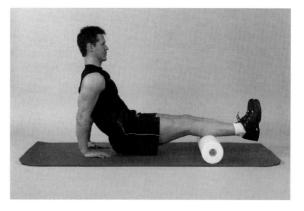

Start seated with your calves on the foam roller. Place your hands directly below your shoulders for maximum stability. Using your arms for leverage, lift your hips off the floor and roll your calves along the foam roller.

Roll from the area above your Achilles tendon to just below your knee. If you find a tight spot, hold that spot and point your toes up and down to stretch that region. To intensify, cross one leg over the other and press down with the top leg.

Variation

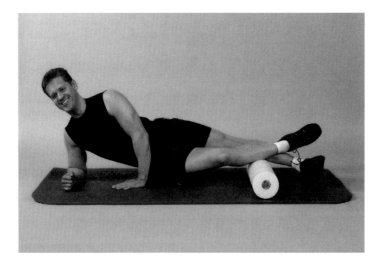

This variation is very effective at accessing the medial (inside) calf muscles along the lower leg. Place your left calf onto the foam roller and turn your torso to the right. Roll along the calf applying pressure along the inside of your shin bone. Pressure should not be applied to the bone itself. Repeat for the other side.

Exercises

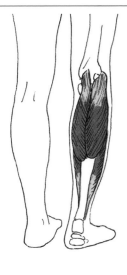

Note: To set yourself up for the stretches described below, position an OPTP Slant™ 1 - 2 feet away from a wall (if needed for support). Bend your right knee and let your pelvis shift forward. (If you're using a wall for support do not push against it.) The stretch should be felt in your right leg and your heel should remain in contact with the Slant™ during the stretch. (This stretch can be peformed without the Slant™, but the intensity will be less.)

To focus on the gastroc-nemius muscle, keep your right leg straight. A stretch should be felt in the upper part of the calf. Repeat for the left side.

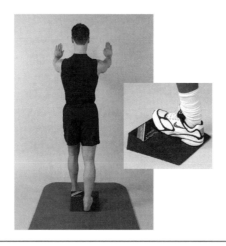

To focus on the soleus muscle, slowly bend your right knee. A stretch should be felt in the lower portion of the calf. Repeat for the left side.

Stretches

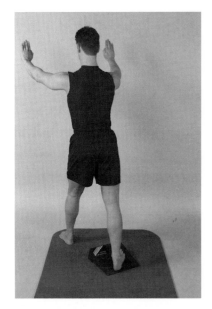

To focus on the Achilles tendon, position the Slant™ so that it's rotated 45 degrees counter-clockwise. Perform the soleus stretch shown above, but instead step toward your left with your left foot and face it forward. This will focus the stretch on your right Achilles tendon.

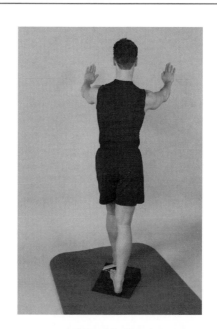

Reposition the Slant™ 45 degrees clockwise and step to your right with your left foot to stretch the inside of your right Achilles tendon. Repeat both stretches for the left side.

36

Lower Legs

shin (anterior tibialis muscles)

Foam Roller Massage

Tools Needed: 36" x 6" Foam Roller

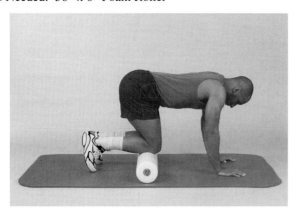

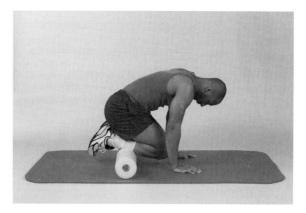

Place both shins on the foam roller and allow your body weight to fall to both your shins and hands.

Roll from below your knees to your ankles. Be careful not to roll directly on the bony portion of your shin.

Variation

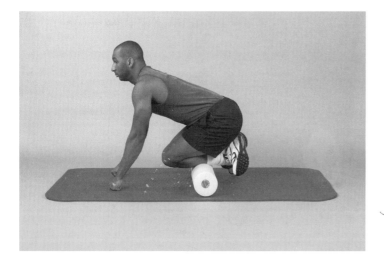

For more intensity, cross one leg over the other to focus on one shin at a time. Again, avoid the bony part of your shin. Repeat for the other leg.

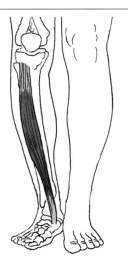

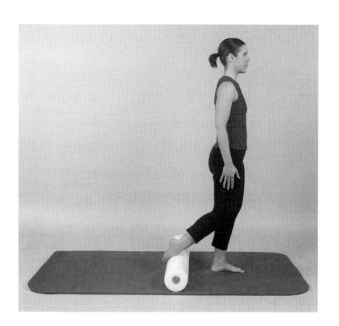

For a standing stretch, bend both knees and place the top of your right foot on the roller. Slowly bend your left knee and lower your body to feel a stretch on the top of your lower right leg. Repeat on the opposite side.

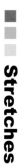

Sit back on your heel keeping the top of your foot flat on the floor. To intensify the stretch, pull up on your forefoot. Repeat on the opposite side.

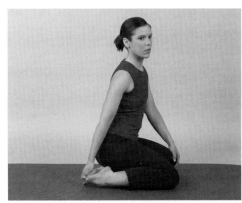

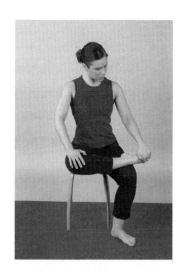

Start seated with your right leg crossed over your left thigh. Clasp your foot with your left hand and slowly pull your foot toward your body without letting your foot turn inward or outward. Repeat on the opposite side.

Stretches

Foam Roller Massage

Tools Needed: 36" x 6" Foam Roller, Stretch Out® Strap

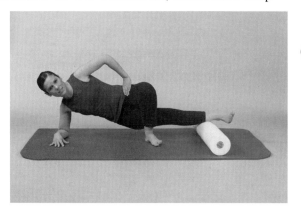

Note: If tingling or numbness is felt in your left leg you may be rolling too close to your knee and the peroneal nerve. This should be avoided.

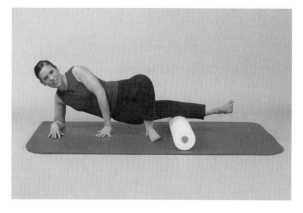

Start side-lying with your right elbow under your right shoulder. Place the side of your right lower leg on the roller and cross your left leg over in front for stability. Raise your hips off the floor and apply pressure to the side of your right leg.

Using your left leg and right arm, slowly roll along your lower right leg between your knee-cap and ankle. Repeat on the opposite side.

Variation

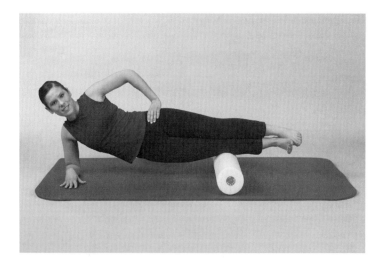

To intensify the massage, increase pressure by placing both legs on the roller and roll along the lower leg. Repeat on the opposite side.

Exercises

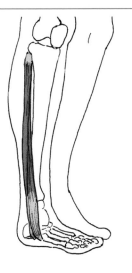

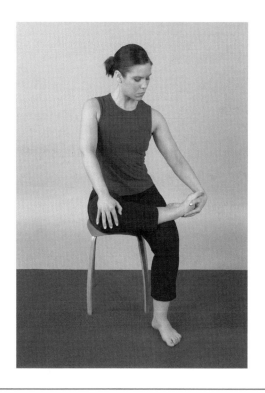

Start seated and cross your right leg over your left thigh. Place the palm of your left hand over the top of your right foot and slightly turn your foot inward. Slowly draw your foot in until a stretch is felt along the outside of your lower leg. Repeat on the opposite side.

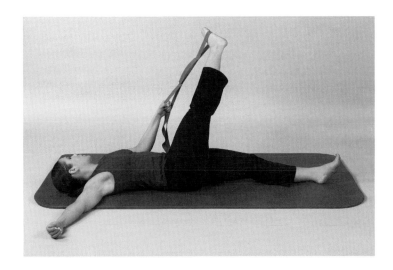

Place the Stretch Out® Strap around the ball of your right foot. Pull the strap toward your torso and allow your right foot to turn inward (pigeon toed). Keep your knee straight, but not locked. A stretch should be felt along the outside of your lower leg and ankle. Repeat on the opposite side.

Stretches

40

Ball Massage

● Tools Needed: Super Pinky massage ball

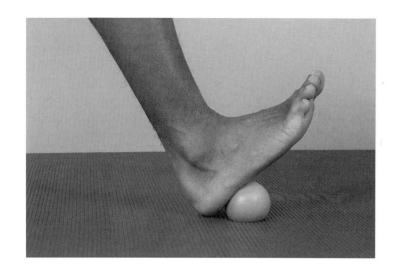

Place a massage ball under your foot. Flex your toes back toward your shin and lower your heel down to the floor.

Exercises

Variation

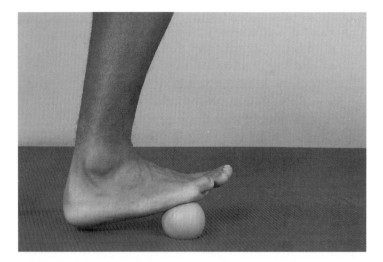

For a dynamic massage of the plantar area, roll from the ball of your foot to your heel while applying downward pressure on the massage ball. Repeat on the opposite side.

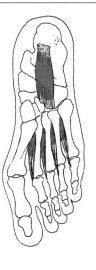

Place your toes up against a wall with the heel and ball of your foot on the floor. Roll your foot side to side without allowing the ball of your foot or heel to leave the floor. Hold positions where tightness is felt. This stretch can be modified by bending and straightening your knee. Repeat on the opposite side.

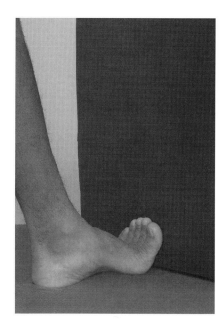

Stretches

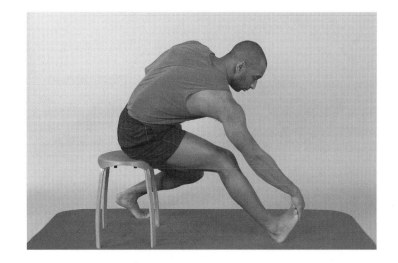

Start seated. Place the palm of your hand over the toes of your foot and pull back until a stretch is felt on the bottom of your foot. Repeat on the opposite side.

Note: If you're unable to touch your toes, loop the Stretch Out® Strap around the ball of your foot and proceed.